Contents

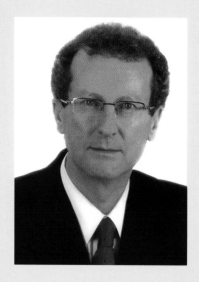

ABOUT THE AUTHOR

Martin Healy studied for three years at the College of Traditional Acupuncture, England, graduating in 1983. A member of the British Acupuncture Council, he trained under Professor J.R. Worsley, who pioneered the use of Five Element Acupuncture.

After graduation Martin Healy studied with Dr. Anthony Hodson, a pioneer researcher into allergy medicine in England. Since then he has worked almost exclusively with allergy patients, and a particular Food Intolerance test. Five Element Acupuncture provides the other dimension of his unique approach.

He now brings this unique experience to the Sam McCauley Chemists organisation and to his own practice in Dublin.

Photographer Edmund Ross

Introduction

In our increasingly, busy world, more and more people - men, women, teenagers and even babies - are suffering from food allergies. We are all familiar with the health warnings associated with the excessive consumption of foods such as salt, fat, sugar etc. However, it is a revelation to many people that the most common allergic foods are those very items which we have been advised are healthiest for us, such as high fibre breakfast cereals, wholemeal bread, calcium-rich dairy products, vitamin-rich citrus fruit and many more. For certain people, allergies to these everyday foods can be the cause of many common medical conditions such as asthma, eczema, arthritis, migraine, sinusitis, irritable bowel syndrome etc.

This book has been written to inform you of a new understanding of allergies based on:

How it is now emerging that the majority of food allergy reactions are delayed, sometimes taking several days to manifest.

This is in stark contrast to what was always believed. It also means that many of the tests which were developed prior to this understanding are now obsolete.

This book details my approach to treating allergies and how it has helped many of my patients over nearly twenty years. It pays particular attention to:

- How and why people become allergic

- The differences between the available allergy tests

- How to increase resistance to allergies.

Martin Healy

CHAPTER 1
THE POTENTIAL OF THIS SYSTEM

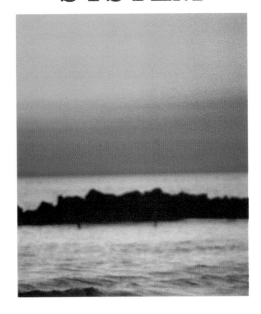

Introduction

It is my belief that many of the illnesses which are presently regarded as medical conditions in themselves - for example, irritable bowel syndrome, asthma, eczema, psoriasis, arthritis, sinusitis, migraine - are in fact nothing more than different mani-festations of the same phenomenon - food allergy. If the allergic foods can be identified accurately and removed from the diet, there is often a significant improvement in health.

Most affected people have relatively few primary allergies - two or three at most - so this process is rarely onerous. Improvement can usually be seen within days of starting, and certainly in less than three weeks.

The following two extracts from recent newspaper articles give an indication of what is possible. They are particularly relevant because the people concerned identified themselves and openly shared with their readers every aspect of their condition, and also the outcome after having the treatment.

The symptoms these articles discuss are the most common presenting symptoms of the majority of allergy sufferers. If your particular complaint is similar to these, it is likely that you can expect a similar outcome.

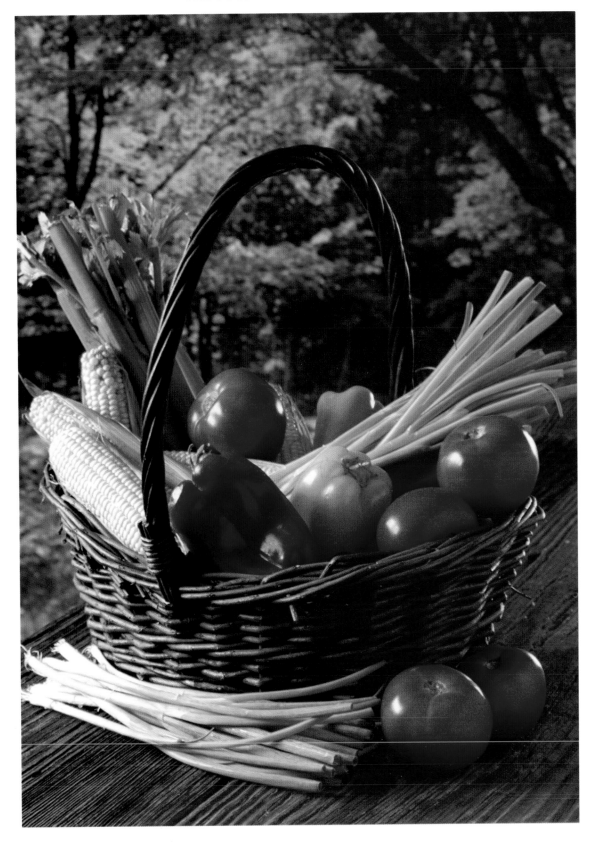

The Big Issue

Rosemarie Meleady* reports on a new procedure, which is set to cause a stir in health circles - a simple allergy test which can quickly identify if you are suffering as a result of food intolerance.

Martin Healy, clinical director of the Fitzwilliam Acupuncture and Allergy Clinic, approached me two months ago about trying out a test he is using to cure people of common complaints such as irritable bowel, eczema, migraine, etc. It was strange because he called on my mother's birthday and the ideal gift for her would be to restore her health.

My mother suffers from severe sinus trouble - by severe I mean she gets up in the morning and starts to sneeze until midday. At around dinner time she would again start to sneeze and could continue sneezing through the night. When I say sneeze, I mean eye-popping forceful sneezes. Often she would sneeze for 48 hours, without hardly a break.

She tried everything, but nothing stopped it. Her face would be constantly swollen, her eyes streamed and the strong medication her GP had her on to suppress the sneezing, would make her sleepy. This had been going on for about twenty years and now that my mother is in her 60s there were

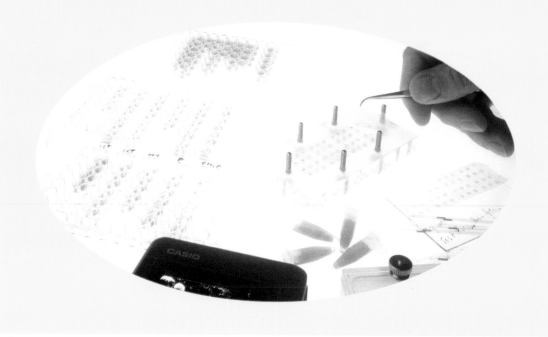

concerns how this constant, exhausting sneezing would affect her heart. She has also suffered from indigestion problems and irritable bowel for as long as she can remember.

So when Healy invited me to send someone on a trial to his clinic I immediately thought of my mother and booked her in.

It took 10 days for my mother's results to come back. The report showed a strong reaction to wheat and yeast, with cows' milk, eggs and legumes (beans and peas) giving a mild reaction. My mother has always made her own bread with wheat germ, bran and all these things which she thought would help her digestion problem when in fact, in her case, these were causing all her health problems.

Three days after ruling these out of her diet she could already see an improvement in her health - she was sleeping much better and wasn't getting her daily bout of indigestion. One week later there were dramatic improvements, with bonuses! Her indigestion had completely gone, she was no longer feeling bloated, she was sleeping much more soundly and the nightmares she experienced nightly since childhood had stopped.

Two weeks after starting the "diet" my mother rang me, exclaiming that for the first time in years she slept breathing through her nose - this may not seem to be a big achievement but it meant she did not wake up with a dry mouth and throat which led to a rasping cough and it also meant that my father was not kept awake by her snoring!

She stopped taking the strong suppressive medication her GP had been prescribing her for 17 years - a month has since passed and she hasn't sneezed once. I now see a different woman - her eyes are no longer puffed, her face has a healthy glow rather than blotchy and swollen and she is of a much healthier weight.

For the first time in her life she could smell the flowers I got her for Mother's Day.

* Rosemarie Meleady is the editor of The Big Issue magazine.*

"The Big Issue" Magazine.

The Irish Times

New allergy tests may mean an end to long lists of forbidden foods - and better results. Already, one Dublin specialist (Martin Healy) is combining them with acupuncture to combat the side effects of the pace of life.

Arminta Wallace was impressed.

(*Irish Times* Journalist)

Why do so many people seem to suffer from allergies nowadays?

Healy says that "the nervous system can be regarded as the intelligence which orchestrates the digestive process. The digestive system is intimately bound up with the emotions - so when the system is subject to persistent heavy doses of stress, it is weakened to the point where it can no longer process certain foods. That's what a food allergy is; it's a food which stays in the gut undigested. The majority of allergy people talk about tummy upsets, bloated feelings, indigestion - these are all triggered by undigested food poisoning the system. And the more we stress and hassle ourselves, the more we weaken the digestive system, to the point where it doesn't recognise and can't process the culprit food."

As for the physical results of all this stress and bother, Healy paints a grim picture. "When food is not digested it begins to curdle and become toxic. If an egg goes off, or milk goes sour, think of how it smells - now think of that inside your body."

This reporter's trial test showed up a fairly serious allergy to dairy products and eggs, something of a shock result for someone who, having been down the irritable bowel/stomach ulcer/early-morning-queasiness road for many years, had taken to drinking vast quantities of milk and eating mountains of scrambled egg in a misguided attempt to improve the digestive situation.

One dairy-free month later the early-morning queasiness has completely vanished and there have been no unpleasant stomach "episodes" at all. No more ice cream, either; but when you feel 100 per cent better, you don't argue with that.

———————

"The Irish Times".

CHAPTER 2
ALLERGY
OR
INTOLERANCE

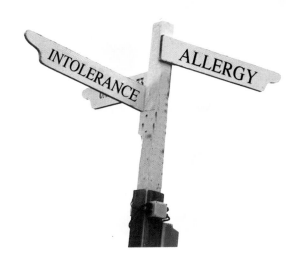

Introduction

Allergies are associated with an imbalance in the immune system. It is a highly complex system but only those aspects which relate to allergies need be discussed here.

Components Of The Immune System

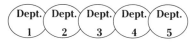

The immune system has several departments, each there to deliver a different kind of defence response. The immune system uses two completely different departments for dealing with allergy-related problems. One triggers diarrhoea or vomiting to flush the allergy intruder out of the body as quickly as possible. The other creates intense inflammation around the allergen in order to incinerate it.

The Immediate Reaction Dept.: triggers the immune system to flush allergens out of the body as quickly as possible.

The Delayed Reaction Dept.: takes a certain time to gather all of the forces of the immune system and then delivers a powerful inflammatory response to allergens which have entered the bloodstream. Consequently, this inflammatory response is delayed. It could take up to two or three days to trigger a reaction. Such delayed reactions are not called allergy but intolerance. These intolerance, delayed-response reactions, are the subject of this book.

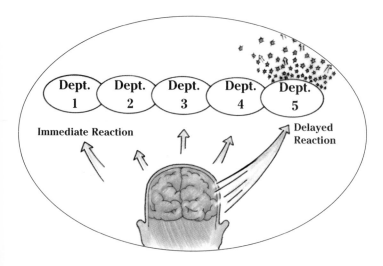

Two Main Types Of Allergy Reaction

The following case histories illustrate the very important differences between immediate and delayed reactions.

Mary (Immediate food allergy reactions)

Mary has had allergy tendencies all her life. As a baby she suffered from colic, and had eczema on her face and hands.

Once, while she was studying for her final examinations at university, Mary became violently sick with vomiting and diarrhoea, her mouth and tongue swelled and she had to be rushed to hospital. This happened immediately after eating a meal in a restaurant. The hospital did an allergy test and diagnosed that she was very allergic to shellfish. Mary realised that she had had prawns as a starter with her lunch and that her tongue had started swelling even before she had finished the main course. She was advised that this type of allergy reaction remains for life and that if ever she ate shellfish again, it was possible that the next reaction could be even more severe. She was also advised to carry a special adrenaline pen so that she could inject herself immediately if ever she found her tongue swelling as a result of inadvertently eating shellfish. By scrupulously avoiding shellfish she has remained well ever since.

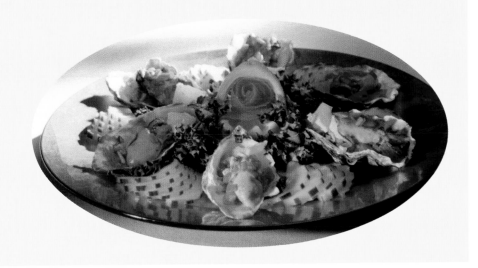

Pat (Delayed food intolerance reaction)

Pat enjoyed very good health for much of his life. Now in his mid-forties, he was appointed manager of a local bank two years ago. For the past year his health has been deteriorating. He has been suffering with irritable bowel syndrome, manifesting as bloating and cramping within the intestines. He is also very tired for much of the time. No matter how much he sleeps, he is never really refreshed for long. His sinus passages are becoming blocked, causing headaches and migraine-type pains across his temples and forehead.

His doctor has tried every investigation possible but nothing specific has shown up. A specialist recommended a high fibre diet for the irritable bowel problem but this only made matters worse. He has a steroid spray for his sinusitis, but it gives only temporary relief and he is also worried about possible long-term effects. He has had three courses of antibiotics already this year for the sinusitis and the relief they give is shorter with each course. In summer his eyes burn and itch and he fears that he is now beginning to suffer with hayfever.

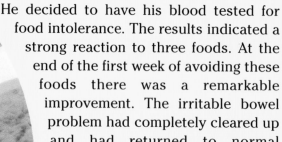

He decided to have his blood tested for food intolerance. The results indicated a strong reaction to three foods. At the end of the first week of avoiding these foods there was a remarkable improvement. The irritable bowel problem had completely cleared up and had returned to normal functioning. By the end of the second week, not alone had the sinusitis cleared but the migraine was almost gone. His energy was back and his zest for life and work had also returned.

Important Differences Between The Two Reactions

There are clear differences between the two food reactions. Mary's allergy, which causes an immediate reaction, is well documented in medical texts and is familiar to the majority of people.

However, the main feature of Pat's intolerance reactions, which made it difficult for his own GP to diagnose, was the fact that he was not showing symptoms immediately after eating the offending foods. The symptoms were building over a period of time as the intolerance foods slowly poisoned his system, causing intense inflammation at various sites. This is "delayed reaction food allergy".

This type of intolerance reaction is rarely discussed in medical texts and is unfamiliar to the majority of people. However, a body of evidence is now emerging which suggests that the majority of foods which trigger reactions, involve the slow poisoning process as described in Pat's case above.

Immediate Allergy Reaction

The most important characteriatic of the Immediate Allergy Reaction is the association of memory with each invader. This type of allergy can produce a more thorough attack on the food with each successive encounter. The great danger with this lies in reactions which produce a swelling of the tongue, lips or the throat. It is very likely that this type of allergy will produce a more severe attack response, with each encounter.

How The Immediate Allergy Reaction Works

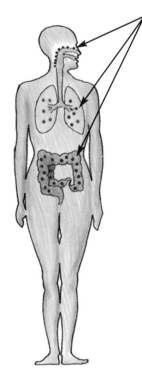

Diagram 1

Mast cells are special sacs which contain protective chemicals. They are embedded in tissues located around the nose, the lungs and in the intestines. *(See Diagram 1).*

At these sites they are well positioned to guard the body's vulnerable entrance points from invaders.

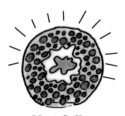

Mast Cell

Once the allergy trigger enters the body, it signals the mast cell to release its chemical contents, causing chaos in the surrounding tissues. One of the main chemicals released is histamine, hence the use of drugs to counteract its effects called antihistamines. Histamine is the hormone which triggers all the classic symptoms of allergy, including:

- coughing and sneezing
- streaming eyes and nose
- vomiting
- diarrhoea
- swelling of the tissues.

All of this represents the body's attempt to get the offending invader out of the body as quickly as possible. The immediate allergy reaction is most commonly triggered by external factors such as dust, pollen, cat or dog hair, parasites etc. Only a small number of foods are known to trigger this reaction.

Because of this immediate reaction, the majority of people are able to recognise their own trigger agents and seldom need to resort to specific allergy tests.

The Delayed Intolerance Reaction

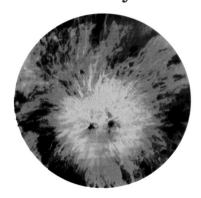

The delayed intolerance reaction is primarily concerned with foods which become toxic within the intestines and make their way into the bloodstream. This time the immune system confronts such toxins and attaches itself to their surface. In this way it attracts the most powerful inflammatory cells of the immune system, directing them to attack whatever it is attached to. Heat and intense inflammation are by-products of the attack.

Predominant Characteristics of the Delayed Intolerance Reaction

- It activates a major defence response.

- It attempts to neutralise the invader by creating intense inflammation in the area concerned.

- The reactions which result from this intolerance response take two to three days to manifest, making it almost impossible for the individual to trace which particular foods are making him or her ill.

Much of the confusion relating to allergies stems from the lack of understanding of this particular slow reaction.

Most allergy tests are designed to detect immediate allergy reactions. Because the majority of foods do not activate the immediate allergy reaction, the tests come back negative. Thus the tendency has been to deny the existence of most food allergies.

Conditions Associated with Food Intolerance

Many of our most common chronic conditions are potentially associated with this delayed intolerance reaction. Conditions where the symptoms of inflammation such as heat, redness, pain, swelling etc., are the outstanding features, and which can not be direcly associated with an injury or obvious infection, should be investigated with this in mind.

Conditions primarily Associated with Food Intolerance:

- Sinusitis
- Indigestion
- Tiredness
- PMT
- Hormone Imbalance
- Bowel Disorders
- Thyroid Disease
- Candida
- Asthma
- Stomach Complaints
- Acne Infections
- Asthma
- Stomach Complaints
- Acne
- Infections
- M.E.
- Skin Problems
- Overweight
- Arthritis

CHAPTER 3
HOW
FOOD
INTOLERANCE
BEGINS

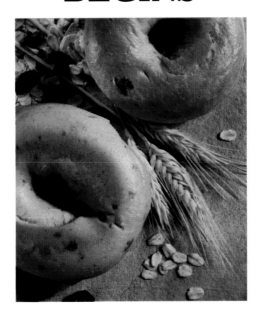

Stress is the Ultimate Cause

The body cannot use any food unless it has first broken it down into its simplest component parts. To do this the digestive glands produce a measured amount of digestive enzyme.

For example : -

• **FATS** trigger the gallbladder to secrete bile in order to dissolve and breakdown the fat as it passes through the digestive system.

• **SUGARS** trigger the insulin glands to produce insulin in order to help with the breakdown and the absorption of sugar as it passes through the system.

The working of the digestive glands is controlled by the nervous system. Worry and stress can overload these nerve pathways, causing the digestive system to malfunction and lose the ability to co-ordinate the proper digestion of food.

This results in undigested foods arriving in the intestines. It is these undigested foods which ultimately become the intolerance foods.

Food Intolerance

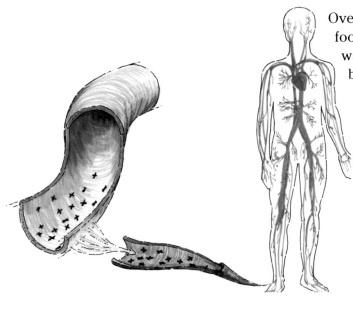

Over time, this build-up of undigested foods and toxins eventually make their way from the bowel into the bloodstream. They are then carried by the blood throughout the body. The immune system responds to this invasion of the blood by activating a delayed intolerance reaction. Heat and intense inflamation are the by-products of this attack.

Symptoms Of Food Intolerance

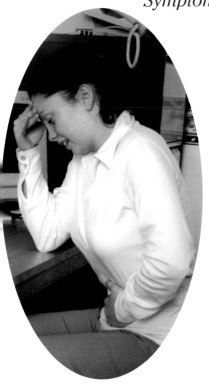

Intestinal upset is common to most food allergy sufferers, other symptoms may include:

- Flatulence and Bloating

- Indigestion

- Diarrhoea or Constipation

- Irritable Bowel Syndrome

- Arthritis

- Skin Conditions

- Sinusitis

- Dandruff or cradle cap in babies

How Food Intolerance Causes Inflammation

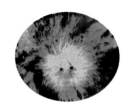

Toxins which originate in the bowel are able to escape into the bloodstream. The immune system responds by triggering the delayed reaction, inflammatory response to destroy them. However, the continuous leakage of toxins from the bowel results in a flood of the most powerful inflammatory cells into the bloodstream to attack them.

The immune system is supposed to direct these inflammatory cells against the toxins. However, the continuous flood of inflammatory cells into the bloodstream results in saturation and this cause the irritation and inflammation of the affected organs and joints.

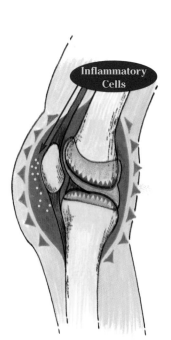

The very same principle applies to eczema, sinusitis, diabetes, irritable bowel syndrome, asthma, migraine etc, and a host of other immune system related conditions. The continuous flood of attack, inflammatory, immune cells into the blood stream is causing saturation and they eventually begin attacking and causing chronic inflammation of the body's own tissues and organ systems.

One example of this:

In this diagram there is a flood of inflammatory cells into the knee joint causing heat, swelling and inflamation.

How To Treat These Conditions

By finding the intolerant foods and eliminating them from your diet, you stop the creation of these bowel toxins. In turn the immune system stops producing these attack, inflammatory, immune cells.

CHAPTER 4
TOXIC
BOWEL

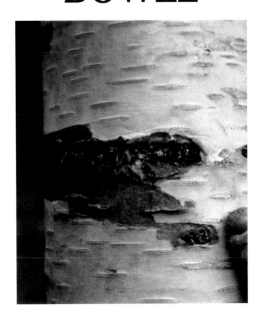

Introduction

The digestive tract is approximately 30 feet long and, in the average adult, contains up to $2^1/_2$ pounds of living bacteria, the majority within the large and small intestines. These bacteria can be thought of as either friendly (health-enhancing) or unfriendly (toxin-producing). In good health there is a balance between the friendly and the unfriendly bacteria. Certain factors disturb this delicate balance and if the unfriendly bacteria overwhelm the friendly and outnumber them, the end result is toxins in the bowel.

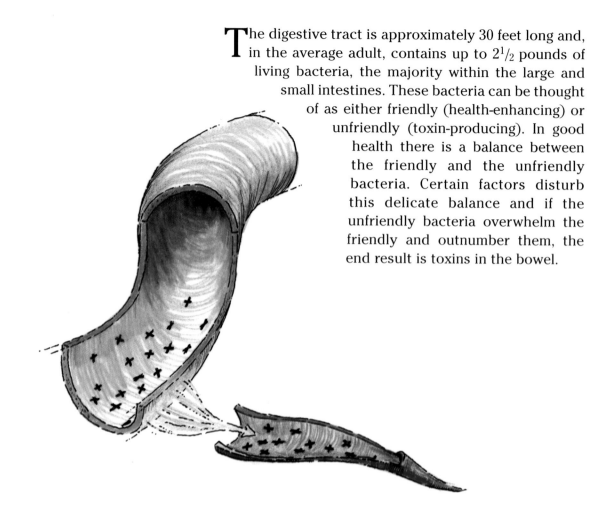

Toxic Bowel

Several factors contribute to the creation of this toxic environment. The biggest contributing factor, however, is food intolerance. These are the foods which arrive in the gut undigested and directly ignite this toxic state within the intestines.

How to Clear the Intestines of Toxic Bacteria

The intestines of people who suffer with food intolerance are overrun with toxic bacteria. The key to resolving all of your problems hinges upon clearing the intestines of these toxins. You have to do three things to remove these toxins:

(1) Diagnose and remove the foods which are feeding these toxic bacteria. The FoodCheck food intolerance test as described in Chapter 12, is the best way to do this.

(2) Ensure complete, daily, bowel evacuation. Sluggish, irregular bowel motions exacerbate all of the food intolerance symptoms. For those who are sluggish, sprinkle one or two dessertspoons of sesame seeds onto your breakfast cereal. Take with warm milk if possible and drink lots of fluids. Sesame seeds are one of the very best aids to thorough bowel evacuation and cleansing.

(3) Use a good probiotic to boost the number of friendly bacteria in your intestines. Seek out a good probiotic and consume daily.

Probiotics

There are many different probiotic products available. For a probiotic to be truly useful and therapeutic it must fulfill certain criteria:

Survive Passage Through Intestinal Tract:

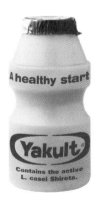

To be effective, a probiotic has to react in the intestines. As survival through the gastrointestinal tract is an essential criterion of a probiotic, it is important that you choose a probiotic that survives the strong gastric acids and other obstacles it has to face along that journey. One such probiotic, Yakult, has numerous randomised, placebo-controlled studies which demonstrate that people given Yakult had an increased count of the beneficial lactobacillus bacteria in their faeces. It also promotes a significant increase in Bifidobacteria counts. This finding is very important because in terms if toxic bowel, the Bifidobacteria are most important in the fight against pathogenic, toxic, gut bacteria.

Safety:

With probiotics, it is vital that the strain of bacteria used, is safe for human consumption. It is essential that the particular bacteria have been adequately tried and tested. The strain of bacteria used in Yakult is guaranteed safe for human consumption.

Potency:

The therapeutic value of a probiotic is determined by the number of live, active bacteria it delivers to the intestines. These probiotic bacteria are delicate and need specialist production techniques to maintain their therapeutic vitality. Trials of some commercially available probiotics have shown them to have inadequate numbers of live, active bacteria. Independent trials have consistently demonstrated that Yakult contains 6.5 billion probiotic bacteria per bottle. This is well in excess of the recommended therapeutic minimum level of 1 billion bacteria.

Milk Base:

For the probiotic bacteria to survive, they need to be cultured in a friendly medium. Milk is the ideal. However, a major problem with using a milk base is that approximately 75% of the people who most need these probiotics, suffer from a dairy intolerance. In such cases the probiotic is actually making matters worse. The milk base is feeding the toxic bacteria in the gut. No benefit is gained from such probiotics. Despite all the current hype and promotion of probiotics, I have found that many of the most popular brands of probiotic, are really making matters worse for the individual concerned.

In my experience it is the fat content of the milk which causes the intolerance reaction, so theoretically, by removing the fat, you remove the problem. Purchasing a probiotic which uses a fermented skimmed milk base (they also have less lactose) can be very effective. There is unlikely to be any negative reactions from the milk and you will gain all of the benefits associated with taking thriving populations of healthy probiotic bacteria.

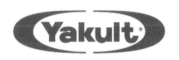 Yakult is a probiotic which uses a fermented skimmed milk base. Yakult is the original probiotic, both in terms of production (first produced 1935) and research.

Bowel Bacteria - A History

Dr. Edward Bach (physician & herbalist) (1886 - 1936)

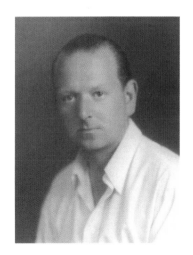

At the turn of the last century Edward Bach, physician, pathologist, bacteriologist and herbalist, recognised that many diseases stemmed from bowel toxicity.

At University College Hospital, London, after many years working in general medicine Bach studied bacteriology. There he discovered that certain intestinal germs, which up until then had been considered of little or no importance, were closely connected with many long-standing and chronic diseases.

He found that particular germs were present in the intestines of all his patients who suffered with chronic disease. Further investigations showed that these same germs were also present in healthy individuals, but were far more prolific in people who were suffering active disease. He began to investigate these bacteria, the relationship they bore to particular diseases and why they were there in such great numbers.

Bach began to understand that the primary cause of this toxicity within the bowel was diet. He noticed that people who ate a healthy diet had very different faeces from those who ate an unhealthy diet. He discovered that there was a definite relationship between the disease condition and the numbers of toxic bacteria present in the bowel. In virtually all cases, as soon as the faecal bacteria start to decline the disease condition starts to disappear. The reverse is also true, in that as soon as the bacterial count starts to increase, the condition begins to worsen.

Bach found that these abnormal bowel bacteria were not in themselves disease-forming. Their danger lies in the toxins which they are slowly producing. It is this prolonged, continued action which gradually and insidiously lowers the vitality of the individual, and this increases the susceptibility to both acute and chronic disease.

Bach writes in his notes of this period that the human subject becomes infected very early in life, and so commonly are these organisms found in adults and children that many laboratories have come to regard their presence as reasonably normal. However, the dramatic improvement in health which is associated with their removal proves that they are far from normal inhabitants.

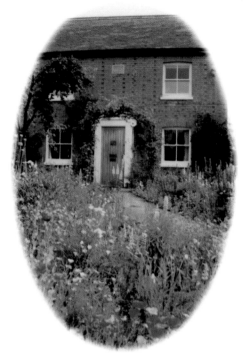

*The Dr. Edward Bach Centre.
Mount Vernon, Sotwell,
Oxfordshire, England*

CHAPTER 5
CANDIDA ALBICANS

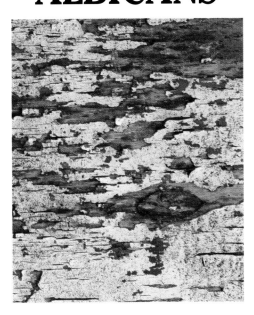

Introduction

There are over four hundred different species of organism within the intestines, of which candida albicans is but one. When it is kept in check by a strong immune system and by flourishing populations of healthy bacteria, candida does not pose a threat to health. A trend has emerged of associating every symptom of intestinal upset and allergy with candida. This is potentially misleading and essentially untrue.

In some people whose immune systems are severely weakened, the candida organism can increase in number within the intestinal tract. As it begins to grow in strength, it develops some characteristics which can pose a serious threat to the health of the individual:

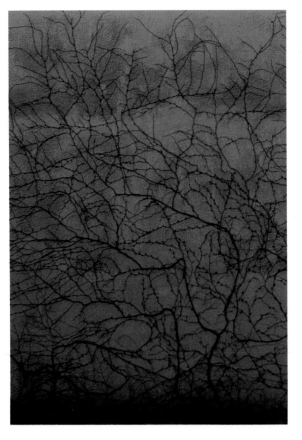

- Candida grows roots which burrow into the intestinal wall, increasing its permeability. The existing toxins within the bowel and the extra toxins which the candida produce are then able to pass more readily into the bloodstream, producing a poisonous state in the body.

- Toxins produced by the candida organism appear to be the most poisonous of all intestinal bacteria.

The Causes Of Candida Overgrowth

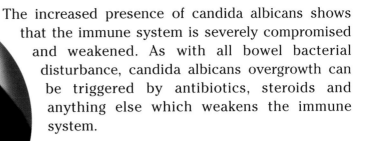

The increased presence of candida albicans shows that the immune system is severely compromised and weakened. As with all bowel bacterial disturbance, candida albicans overgrowth can be triggered by antibiotics, steroids and anything else which weakens the immune system.

Food intolerance is also associated with Candida Albicans. These are the foods which arrive in the gut undigested and directly ignite this toxic state within the intestines.

However, the outstanding feature which I have observed as common to people with a candida problem is extremely high levels of stress, anxiety and worry.

There are specific features characteristically associated with this condition, notably:

- Becoming increasingly sensitive to chemicals. People with yeast overgrowth are often sensitive to cosmetics or perfumes or antiperspirants or any of the other personal care items which we all use, every day of our lives.

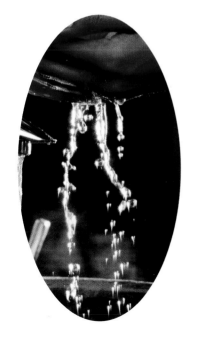

- Worsening of the symptoms in damp weather. Candida albicans is a yeast, and all yeasts thrive in a damp environment. The damper the environment, the more they thrive and the more toxins they produce.

As a result, many people who suffer with Candida Albicans or any other yeast related illness, often experience a noticeable improvement in their general health when they move to a drier climate.

How to Clear the Intestines of Candida Albicans

(1) Use the Food Intolerance test as described in Chapter 12, to diagnose and remove the foods which are feeding the Candida Albicans.

(2) Ensure complete, daily bowel evacuation as described on page 21.

(3) Use a good probiotic to boost the number of friendly bacteria in your intestines. Seek out a good probiotic and consume daily.

Probiotics

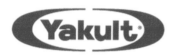

There is an increasing body of evidence from scientific / clinical trials which demonstrates the benefits of consuming probiotics. The most convincing evidence supports the use of probiotics in the treatment of:

- establishing intestinal flora balance
- irritable bowel syndrome
- constipation
- antibiotic associated diarrhoea
- ulcerative colitis and Crohn's disease
- colon cancers
- helicobacter pylori

Note: In addition to the health suggestions in this book, it is imperative that you always seek the expert advice of your own GP.

CHAPTER 6
BABIES
AND
CHILDREN

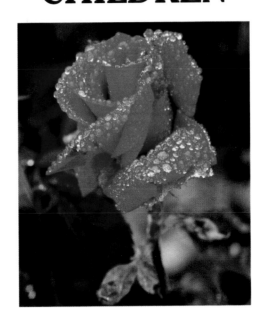

Introduction

This chapter is perhaps the most important in the book because the intolerance approach has the potential to assist many childhood illnesses, quickly and effectively. Many people are unaware that babies and children are very prone to food intolerance but, if the offending allergic food can be found and eliminated from the diet, their improvement is often very dramatic.

Babies' Intestinal Flora

Unlike adults, in whom the balance between friendly and unfriendly bacteria in the gut is reasonably stable, intestinal flora in infants and children can very easily be disturbed. When the unfriendly bacteria dominate, toxins quickly appear, triggering many childhood diseases.

For the majority of adults the bowel wall is an efficient barrier preventing undigested foods and bowel toxins from escaping from the intestines into the bloodstream. However, during the first few weeks of an infant's life, their intestines are very porous.

Because of the porous nature of babies' intestines, undigested food or bacteria can easily make their way into their bodies. This makes babies prime candidates for developing food allergies and sensitivities and marks the beginning of many childhood illnesses. The porousness of babies' intestines normally changes within the first four weeks, but can take up to six months.

Consequently the timing of weaning, when solid foods are introduced, is very important. There is no universally correct time to introduce solid foods. A gradual introduction of new foods is the best approach. Observant parents who are aware of the potential of food intolerance may be able to associate a decline in their child's health with the introduction of a particular new food.

Pregnancy

Food intolerance has a strong hereditary association, appearing to be handed down from parent to child. The chances of a child developing food intolerance appears to be dramatically increased if both parents suffer with food intolerance.

Pregnancy is a critical time in the development of food intolerance. It is very important that food intolerant-prone mothers abstain from any food to which they are sensitive during pregnancy, so that resultant toxins will not reach the developing baby through the blood supply in the placenta.

How To Assist Your Baby Further

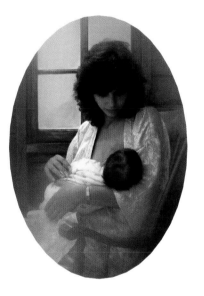

- **Natural Birth:** Bifidobacteria and other friendly micro-organisms enter the babies' intestines as they pass through the birth canal. Babies delivered by Caesarean section have a reduced level of infiltration by these friendly micro-organisms.
- **Breast feeding:** Breast-fed babies have a lower incidence of colic and other digestive disturbances than bottle-fed babies. This is attributed to friendly bacteria (bifidobacteria) whose growth is intensified by mother's milk. These beneficial micro-organisms account for up to 99% of healthy breast-fed babies' intestinal flora.
- **Long Term Feeding:** Long-term breast feeding brings added protection for the child. Feeding for less than 13 weeks results in babies suffering similar rates of intestinal problems as bottle-fed children .

When Breast Feeding Can Be Problematic

The only time when breast feeding is contra-indicated is when the mother herself suffers with food intolerance. What appears to happen is that the mother's own intolerance and associated antibodies make their way into her milk and this upsets the child. When babies who are being breast fed begin to develop conditions which may be allergy related, such as colic, eczema, middle ear infections etc, the mother should be tested for food intolerance first.

I have observed that once a breast-feeding mother has dealt with her own food intolerance, her milk improves and her baby generally settles.

Conditions Affecting Babies and Children

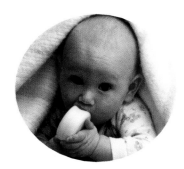

It is my opinion that many of the common conditions of babies and children, including middle ear infections, asthma, eczema, colic, ENT problems etc, are strongly associated with food intolerance. In the majority of cases, the standard treatment is either steroids or antibiotics. For most children, one short course of either does not do any particular harm. The real problems arise when the first course does not work and the child is subjected to repeat courses. Another scenario occurs when the treatment works for a short while but, within a few weeks or months, the child is again ill with the same condition. These are the circumstances in which allergy testing should definitely be considered in order to save the child from becoming debilitated by repeat courses of antibiotics and steroids.

What happens is that the antibiotic kills off the infection but because the underlying cause, the food intolerance, is never resolved, it continues to create toxins which cause further infection and, as a result, the child continuously falls victim to illness. If anything, the repeated use of antibiotics or steroids disturbs the child's delicate bowel bacteria even further and renders him or her more vulnerable to infection.

The majority of children will eventually outgrow their allergies. However, the longer the undiagnosed allergy is allowed to continue and the more medication the child is given to treat the associated illnesses, the slower the child will be to outgrow the food intolerance.

Hyperactivity In Children

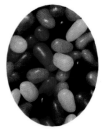

Dr. Ben Feingold was one of the first people to bring attention to the possibility of some hyperactive children being affected by food additives and colourings. However, there is also an association between hyperactivity and intolerance to everyday foods such as eggs, dairy products, meat, bread etc.

Babies not Sleeping at Night

Difficulty in getting the baby off to sleep is another strong indicator of food intolerance.

The Daily Mail

By **Lesley Turney.**

Henny Hind discovered that allergic reactions to a multitude of common substances were at the root of her son's physical and emotional problems.

"As a toddler, Reiner suffered from recurring chest infections and severe eczema. He was hyperactive and had difficulty with sleep and concentration," says Henny. "I was already concerned about the amount of medication he was taking, when someone suggested he might be sensitive to foods, so I decided to have him tested."

It transpired that Rainer was sensitive and I removed all the intolerance foods from his diet straight away. "The eczema cleared up immediately and he had fewer and fewer infections until, a few months later, he became a perfectly healthy, happy, relaxed young boy."

(Reproduced with kind permission of The Daily Mail)

Childhood Conditions which Respond Well to Food Intolerance Testing:

- Hyperactivity
- Sleep disturbance
- Ear infections
- Stomach and intestinal upset
- Asthma
- Skin problems (especially eczema)
- Recurring infections

East Leeds Weekly News

Egg allergy is cracked.
Twins Benjamin and
Thomas Garnett, who
doctors discovered have
an allergy to egg white.
By **Sheila Holmes.**

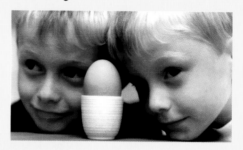

Since they were a week old, identical Leeds twins Benjamin and Thomas Garnett have been plagued with persistent ear infections. Their mother Deborah has taken the boys back and forth to the doctor, the paediatrician and the hospital for the past six years.

But despite having five operations to insert grommets to try to stop their constant pain, the twins did not grow out of the problem as promised, their hearing deteriorated and their temperaments worsened.

Finally Deborah decided to take them for a Food Intolerance test and it was discovered that the twins had identical severe sensitivities.

And just 10 days after changing their diet, Deborah could see a noticeable improvement in the health of both the boys. She said: "Ever since they were babies the boys would cry and scream at night and were very unsettled."

"It was extremely worrying to watch the boys go through the operations at such a young age. Both Tom and Ben have had far more antibiotics than the average child has. I knew that something must be causing their infections, but I could not pinpoint what it was."

"Now they are more confident and much happier. Overall they look healthier, they behave much better and I can only assume that this is because they feel so much better."

Both boys, who had not put on weight for a number of months, have now reached their correct weight, their hearing has improved, the ear infections have gone, the congestion in their sinuses has gone and they have stopped snoring at night.

(East Leeds Weekly News)

CHAPTER 7
WHEAT

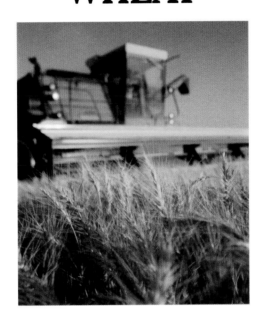

Introduction

Next to dairy products, wheat is the second most common problem food. For the majority of people with a wheat intolerance, total avoidance is impossible and in most cases, not necessary. By avoiding the most problematic parts of the wheat you will experience a dramatic improvement in your general health and still be able to enjoy some wheat products. Equally, the small amounts of wheat used to thicken soups and gravies will normally not affect people. The only people who must totally avoid all wheat products are those with a +4 reaction on the wheat test result. The test grades the degree of intolerance to food on a +1, +2, +3 and +4 scale. A +4 test result on wheat indicates that the person has to avoid wheat completely. However, the new FoodCheck, Food Intolerance test indicates that very few people suffer with +4 intolerance to wheat.

Food Intolerance

The term "food intolerance" in fact means that every person has a certain tolerance level for the particular food. If you do not exceed your tolerance level, the food will not affect you. Equally, it is certain aspects of the food or certain types of processing which renders the food more likely to trigger a reaction. With wheat flour we know that the problematic wheat is the highly processed white flower.

Highly processed white bread is to be totally avoided. Use a good quality light brown sliced bread. Use only the half size loaf as these tend to be more completely baked. The large size loaf is sometimes less well baked and the doughy centre of the loaf increases the intolerance factor. Many highly processed white breads have this high doughy intolerance factor.

Recommended Bread:

There are many good quality light brown sliced breads on the market. One that I particularly like is the Hovis Butterkrust brown loaf. It comes in a bright yellow wrapper.

Another company is the LifeFibre Bread Company who produce a range of quality bread. They incorporate additional healthy ingredients into their breads. These additional ingredients range from apricot and sesame seed to oat bran and linseeds. Many of these extra ingredients bestow additional health giving properties to these breads.

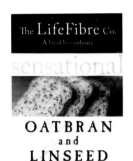

OATBRAN
and
LINSEED
bread

The soluble fibre aspect of oatbran is by far the superior bran to add to bread. This soluble fibre helps to keep your colon environment clean and healthy. The linseeds and sesame seeds also assist with thorough bowel evacuation. The addition of seeds reduce the GI index score of the bread making it an ideal bread for anyone interested in eating breads which will help them to loose weight. The GI index weight loss principle is explained in chapter 14.

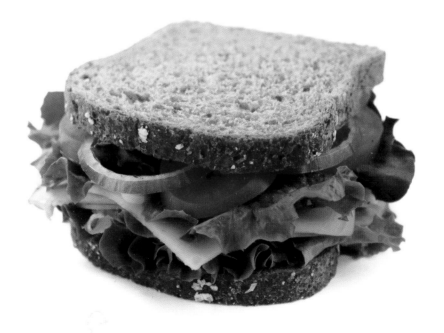

The Ideal Breakfast Cereal

Cereals have always played a great part in human nutrition and oats, more than any of the others, have the greatest nutritional value with many health giving benefits. Porridge is a natural wholegrain - unlike refined grains which have some of the components removed. Wholegrain products include the bran, the germ and the endospern. It has been suggested that all the constituents in the grain act in concert to produce their significant health benefits.

There are many reasons why I continuously recommend porridge but in the contexts of this book, the first relates to the fact that it so very rarely causes any form of food intolerance reaction.

Porridge is light on the stomach because the starch contained in oats is particularly easy to digest. This makes it an ideal starter food in the morning. Porridge is warming and fills you up, especially on cold winter mornings. Try making your porridge with skimmed milk. It makes for a creamy, more nutritious meal and add honey as a sweetener if required. It digests slowly and effortlessly and this in turns produces a slow, gradual, controlled rise in blood sugar levels, just as nature designed.

It has a low GI index (refer to GI chapter) which means that it keeps you going and feeling full for longer. The low GI index also means that it is an ideal food to incorporate into any weight loss programme.

Because it is light on the stomach and easy to digest, it is an ideal night time snack before going to bed. It will never give you that "heavy stomach" feeling the next morning as eating sandwiches or cakes late at night so often does.

- Porridge oats is one of those few foods that contain a high level of soluble fibre which can help to reduce cholesterol.

- You could dramatically increase your soluble fibre intake by simply adding just one tablespoon of oat bran to the oat cereal mix before cooking.

- The fibre in oats is the best form of fibre for people who suffer with food intolerance problems and will not irritate a sensitive colon. A high fluid intake is important to complement the action of this high fibre food. A fluid intake of 6-8 glasses is recommended each day.

- Porridge oats are low in sugar, fat and salt.

Organic Oats

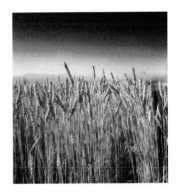

Organic agriculture uses systems that promote the environmentally sound production of wholesome food. Use a 100% organic porridge product which is certified by the Organic Trust.

Flap Jacks

Nutritious oaty flap jacks make for an ideal snack bar. These Flap Jacks are a combination of fruit combined with the natural goodness of oat flakes.

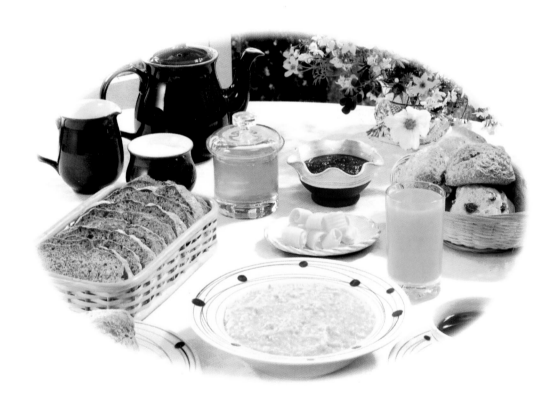

CHAPTER 8
DAIRY PRODUCTS

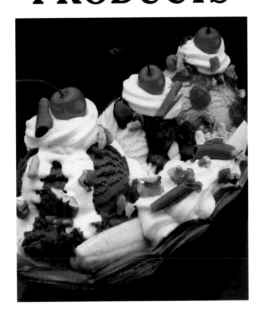

Introduction

One food source which deserves special attention is dairy products. Allergy books are generally either totally for or totally against dairy products. My own personal view is that if you can digest milk, it perhaps is one of the finest and most nutritious foods available. If, on the other hand, you are eating dairy products and your body cannot digest them, they are perhaps one of the most toxic, as even small amounts can trigger serious illness in senstitive people.

Why Is Milk The Most Common Allergy Food?

Of all of the foods which are available to us, milk is perhaps the most complete. It has virtually everything which is required to sustain life. For the first few months of our lives we are able to survive on milk alone. However, because it is such a concentrated food it requires strong digestion to break it down. By contrast, simpler foods such as potato, carrot, rice etc are much easier to digest and rarely cause problems.

Putrefacation

When plant matter which is poorly digested passes through the digestive system, it decays with very few undesirable by-products. However, when dairy products which are not properly digested pass through the system, they putrefy within the gut. The putrefacation process produces a number of undesirable toxic by-products which cause the illnesses associated with dairy senstitivity.

Calcium and Osteoporosis

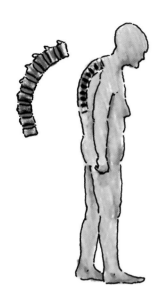

The heated debate which often centres around the suggestion of avoiding dairy products stems from the fear of losing body calcium levels and, as a result, developing osteoporosis. However, the reality of food intolerance is that the body cannot tolerate or process that particular food. Having a dairy intolerance means that you can not process the dairy product, which in turn means that you can not extract the calcium from it. What has been happening with many women who are now suffering with osteoporosis is that they have been depending on and, in many cases, taking extra, dairy products, to increase their calcium levels in the hope of preventing osteoporosis. However, because they have been allergic to the dairy products, they have not been extracting the calcium. Most women with a confirmed diagnosis of osteoporosis are in fact suffering with a dairy products intolerance.

Alternative To Cows' Milk

As has been stated throughout this book, allergy and intolerance are completely different. Anyone with a milk allergy must avoid milk completely. Less than 2% of the population suffer with true milk allergy. However, a large percentage of people suffer from a degree of milk intolerance. Milk intolerance means that you have a degree of difficulty with digesting milk.

It was always assumed that the lactose was the problematic part of the milk. This is incorrect. The majority of supposed lactose intolerant people thrive on either skimmed or goats milk. Yet both skimmed milk and goats milk contain lactose. The reality is that it is the fat content which causes the intolerance reaction. Remove the fat content and you will then be able to digest the milk without difficulty. Additionally, you will be able to absorb all of the many nutrients within the milk including the essential calcium.

Skimmed milk is not suitable for babies or very young children but is suitable for most children over 5 years of age. Always seek the advice of a suitably qualified practitioner.

Skimmed milk will dramatically assist slimmers. This one, simple, dietary change has transformed the lives of many of my chronically, overweight patients. Another health benefit associated with the use of skimmed milk is that it can help lower blood cholesterol. Changing to skimmed milk dramatically reduces the rate of plaque build-up around your teeth. These are but a few of the many health benefits associated with a change to skimmed milk.

Full fat milk camouflages the distinctive taste of the many exotic coffee and tea drinks now available to us. Drink tea with added skimmed milk and you will actually taste the tea. There are many coffee shops throughout the country and most are now willing to make you a coffee using skimmed milk. Try it and note how you can actually taste the coffee. Skimmed milk is better to quench your thirst. With the fat removed from the milk you will not get that fat taste or fat coating in your mouth. With the fat removed your mouth feels more refreshed afterwards. It takes about two weeks to get used to the new taste of skimmed milk but after that, you will wonder how you ever beforehand drank full fat milk.

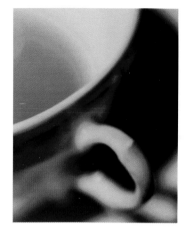

Nutritionally, skimmed milk is equal to standard milk and in many cases has a higher nutrient content. Skimmed milk has a higher protein and calcium content. For example, the calcium content of standard full fat milk is 118mg / 100ml serving. The calcium content of skimmed milk is 136mg / 100ml serving.

Calcium Supplements

I recommend a daily calcium supplement for everyone with a dairy intolerance. Choose a calcium supplment with added Vitamin D as this assists the absorbtion of calcium. Avoid calcium supplements which have many additional vitamins and minerals added to their calcium formula. Such complex combinations may irritate your system. Take calcium supplements with food and never on an empty stomach. Ask your pharmacist for advice with regard to choosing the very best calcium product available.

Alternative to Butter

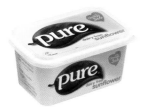

People with a milk intolerance must avoid butter. Some spreads which are now promoted as a butter replacement contain hydrogenated oils. Such products are detrimental to your health and must be totally avoided. The whole Pure range is dairy free. They contain:

- No hydrogenated oils
- Virtually trans-fat free
- They are high in essential polyunsaturated oils and low in saturated fat
- Pure sunflower contains omega 3 and 6 oils.

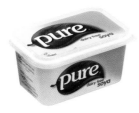

It is altogether an excellent product range.

Note: If Pure spread is not available at your local supermarket, speak with the store manager.

View the table below to find out which Pure spread is perfect for you and your dietary needs.

	Pure Soya	Pure Sunflower	Pure Organic
Free from			
Dairy	✓	✓	✓
GM ingredients	✓	✓	✓
Hydrogenated oils	✓	✓	✓
Artficial additives	✓	✓	✓
Gluten	✓	✓	✓
Soya		✓	
Contains			
Less than 1% salt	✓	✓	
Folic acid	✓	✓	
Omega 3+6		✓	
Vitamin D	✓	✓	✓
Vitamin E	✓	✓	
Vitamin A	✓	✓	✓
Vitamin B12	✓	✓	
Vitamin B6	✓	✓	
Other benefits			
Certified by the Soil Association			✓
Suitable for cooking	✓	✓	✓
Suitable for baking	✓	✓	✓

Alternative to Chocolate

Lindt Excellence

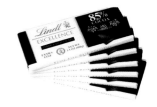

People who suffer with an intolerance to dairy products are often heartbroken at the thought of having to avoid chocolate. It is the nations' favourite snack food. The good news is that cocoa based chocolate eaten in moderation, will not cause food intolerance reactions.

The evidence is mounting that dark chocolate with a high cocoa content, contains chemicals believed to help lower the risk of heart disease. Trials are still continuing but if successful, we could see doctors recommending a few squares of dark chocolate per day as part of a healthy diet.

Green & Black's

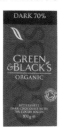

The benefit stems from the cocoa which is a powerful antioxidant and has the ability to neutralise dangerous chemicals in the body. It is also thought to have blood-thinning capabilities, and thus reducing the chances of developing a clot. Is thought to help dilate constricted blood vessels and clear fat deposits which clog the arteries.

A Word Of Caution To Vegetarians

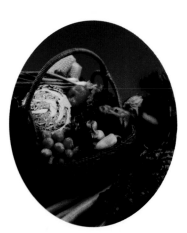

People who do not eat meat often rely on dairy products for their protein and other essential nutrients, so problems arise when vegetarians become sensitive to dairy products. It is my opinion that the vegetarian approach in such cases is not to be recommended. The diet becomes too restricted and the potential of developing nutritional deficiencies becomes a real possibility.

CHAPTER 9
OSTEOPOROSIS

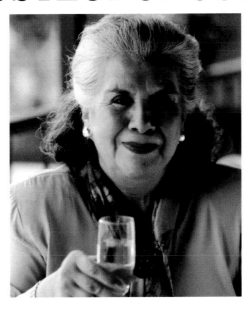

Introduction

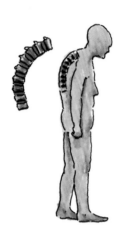

The average woman has achieved maximum bone strength by the age of 25 to 35, after which it begins to leak away. Osteoporosis means literally "porous bones". It is a disease in which the bones become very porous , increasingly fragile, and prone to easily breaking. It shows no outward signs, however, until it is firmly established. Osteoporosis can affect the whole skeleton but more commonly causes vulnerability in spine, hip and wrist bones.

Many women suffering with osteoporosis arrive at menopause with the condition well established. In a lot of cases the condition has started many years beforehand. Once menopause begins, these women then experience an increase in the rate of loss of bone mineral density which is more than the average. This accelerated loss continues for a period of about five years.

Key Factors In The Prevention of Osteoporosis

- Calcium is a major component of the building blocks of bone. Dairy products are the number one source of calcium for the majority of people; yet intolerance to dairy products is almost endemic in Western societies. If you have an intolerance to dairy products you will extract no calcium from them. The new FoodCheck, Food Intolerance test is the best way to be certain whether you are intolerant to dairy products or not.

- As described above, the link between hormone imbalance and osteoporosis is very strong. Symptoms such as pre-menstrual tension (PMT) and other hormone associated symptoms, all indicate a degree of hormone imbalance or hormone sensitive and should not be neglected.

- Regular exercise is an essential factor in maintaining good general health; but it is especially important for maintaining healthy bone structure.

Test for Osteoporosis

Osteoporosis gives no warning signals. It often takes a sudden or unexpected fracture to highlight the reality that the condition is well established. Once bone density has been severely lost, it is very difficult to re-establish the same bone strength.

So it is vital to diagnose this condition as early as possible. The only way to confirm this is to have a diagnostic x-ray test. Measurements are then taken every two or three years to track your progress.

Another Excellent Diagnostic Test

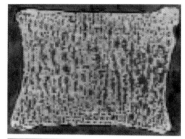
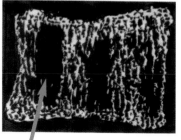

Bone disintegration

Another excellent diagnostic test is known as the NTx Bone Resorption Market Test. This test measures the rate at which you are shedding bone cells. Old bone cells are excreted from the body in urine. The test is a very specific marker of bone disintegration and one which the laboratory can very accurately measure. When there are increased amounts of Ntx in the urine, there is an increased rate of bone destruction.

If you are diagnosed with osteoporosis you will need to begin a course of treatment immediately. Once you begin treatment you will need to know if the treatment is working.

This test tells you what is happening to your bones on any given day, and whether the accelerated bone loss has stopped. Equally it can tell you if the bone loss is continuing and if so, whether it is very slow or at an alarming rate.

No other diagnostic test gives such an accurate account of what is happening to your bones. It permits you to assess your progress as a result of treatment over a short space of time.

All you have to do is collect a very small, mid stream urine sample. The sample is sealed in a special container and posted back for analysis at the laboratory. The results of the analysis will be posted to you.

For details of how to order the NTx Bone Resorption Marker test refer to the Order Form page at the back of this book.

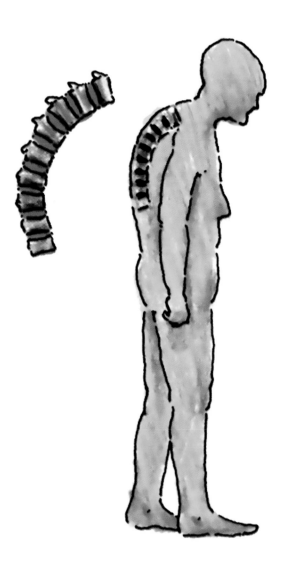

CHAPTER 10
FEMALE HORMONES

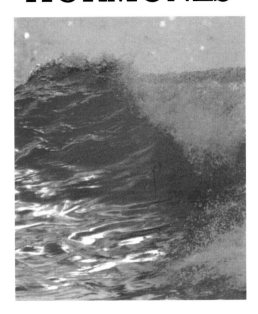

Introduction

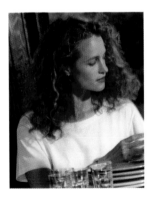

There are a number of medical problems specific to women, from osteoporosis to PMT, which are associated with degrees of imbalance within the female hormonal system.

The female hormones, oestrogen and progesterone, work together as a pair. Oestrogen stimulates many of the female body systems and progesterone protects these systems from over-stimulation, In particular, excessive oestrogen over-stimulates breast and uterine lining.

How HRT Is Supposed To Help

The female hormone oestrogen has many functions within the body:

- Helps to keep healthy many tissues within the body e.g. skin, lining of the vagina, urinary system
- Maintains normal menstrual cycle
- Prevents thinning of the bones.

During the menopause oestrogen levels begin to decrease. As the level of oestrogen falls, symptoms relating to many of its functions begin to develop. HRT uses artificial oestrogen and progesterone to reduce the symptoms of this hormonal decline.

However, there are many continuing doubts about its safety, especially in the long-term.

The Mistake Made

Some women have problems taking HRT because they are rarely, if ever, tested to assess their exact hormone levels. It is instead prescribed in standard doses and its appropriateness assessed on whether it causes side-effects or not. Side-effects, however, can take between six months and two years to appear and, because of the time delay, are not then associated with the HRT.

Regular measurement of hormone levels would avoid all these problems.

Natural Progesterone

Menpoausal decrease in oestrogen is estimated to be approximately 60%, whereas progesterone depletion can be 100%. As a result of this new understanding of hormonal levels, many preactitioners are now not prescribing HRT but instead are prescribing natural progesterone.

Much of this work is based upon the lifetime study of Dr. John Lee. However, the sad reality is that the same mistake made with HRT, is being repeated with natural progesterone. The progesterone levels are not being monitored. Natural progesterone is a very potent hormone and if not monitored, quickly reaches saturation level. Such elevated levels of progesterone suppress the immune system.

How to Test Your Own Hormone Levels

Blood Tests

Blood tests are used to measure hormone levels, but these have disadvantages. Of the total number of hormones in your bloodstream, only a very small number of free hormones, between 1% and 10% are of benefit to the body at any given time. The majority are in a form that the body cannot use (bound hormones). Blood tests record your overall hormone levels but are unable to advise how much of that is of any use to you. Given that some of these hormones are measured in one-billionth of a gram (equivalent to a pinch of salt in a swimming-pool), you can see how precise a successful hormone test needs to be.

The New Saliva Test

There is a much better way of testing for oestrogen and progesterone hormone levels. Only those hormones which can breakout and penetrate the tissues are of any real use to you. These free, unbound hormones also enter into your saliva and can easily be measured there.

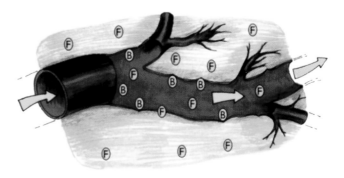

(F) Free unbound hormones

(B) Bound hormones

A major advantage of the saliva test has to do with the ability to collect the sample over a 2-hour period. The reason for this is that sex hormones are produced in "spurts", over a period of hours. The oestradiol, for example, spikes a number of times. If a patient collects the sample at one point in time it is possible for them to produce a sample which is not representative of the hormone being produced for that day.

Blood tests can only be taken at hospitals, clinics or GP surgeries, at an appointed time.

Saliva testing is done in the privacy of your own home. A small saliva sample is collected over a 2-hour period. This is then posted to the clinic for analysis.

Your results
The report that you will receive will tell you what your oestrogen and progesterone levels are. It will clearly show your hormone levels in relation to a recommended range..

Pregnancy

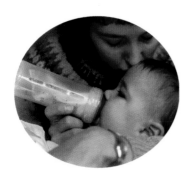

Every woman who is attempting to becomg pregnant, but is experiencing ongoing disappointment and difficulty, should firstly check her hormone status. Nothing will happen for her if she is suffering from a major hormone imbalance. The saliva hormone test is the ideal starting point for a woman experiencing such disappointment.

> **To order the saliva test: refer to Order Form page at the back of this book.**

How to Treat Hormone Imbalance

The intestines of women who suffer with hormone imbalance are very often prone to a degree of disturbance of their gut bacteria. Toxins which originate in the intestines are able to escape into the bloodstream where they cause irritation and inflammation of the ovaries. This on-going inflammation ultimately leads to hormone imbalance.

(1) Use the Food Intolerance test as described in Chapter 12, to diagnose and remove the foods which are feeding these intestinal toxins.

(2) Of the herbal treatments available, Black Cohosh appears to be effective for some women. It has a particularly good record in relation to alleviating some of the symptoms associated with the menopause. Adverse effects are extremely uncommon and no known significant adverse drug interactions.

It is however, contraindicated in pregnancy. It is for short-term use only (maximum of six months) as no studies are available to assess its safety in the long-term.

(3) Many of the symptoms associated with menopause respond extremely well to natural progesterone. However, these creams are very potent and should only be used under the supervision of your GP. Additionally, it is imperative that you use the saliva test to ensure your hormone levels remain within the recommended range.

(4) Classical acupuncture is another option as it is very effective in assisting with all manner of infertility, menopause and other hormone related problems. It is side effect free and very fast acting. Many women feel significantly better within five to six treatments and definitely worth considering.

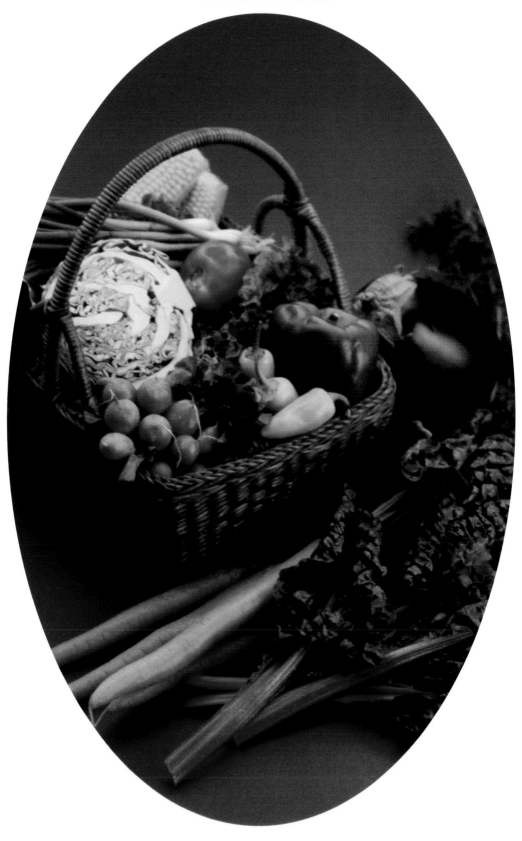

CHAPTER 11
CHOLESTEROL

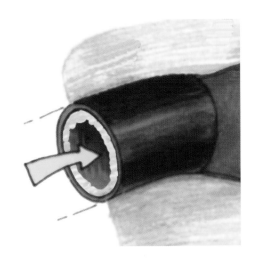

Introduction

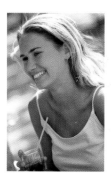

Coronary heart disease is one of the biggest killers in the country. It has traditionally been considered a man's disease, and so it is, but it is also a leading cause of death among women. Before the onset of the menopause, women enjoy a significant degree of protection from heart disease. However, after the menopause, death rates as a result of heart disease jump dramatically. Overall, approximately 20% of female deaths in Ireland are associated with heart disease.

Coronary Heart Disease

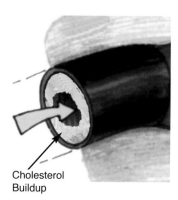

Cholesterol
Buildup

In order to work properly, your heart needs a constant supply of oxygen. The oxygen is carried in the blood, which flows through the coronary arteries to the heart muscle. Coronary heart disease is the term used to describe what happens when this supply is blocked. It is caused by a build up of fatty substances (cholesterol) in the arteries. If the coronary arteries become partially blocked, this can lead to chest pains called angina. If the arteries become completely blocked, this can lead to a heart attack.

According to some estimates, nearly half of all heart disease deaths are due to high cholesterol levels. Yet it is estimated that seven out of ten people are above the recommended limits of 5.0mmol. There are two types of cholesterol, one good and the other bad.

Bad Cholesterol

The bad one is known as LDL cholesterol. It dumps fat into the arteries, where it starts to narrow the gap through which the blood supply can pass. Once the artery gets completely blocked, a heart attack occurs.

Good Cholesterol

Good cholesterol is known as HDL and it removes fat from the arteries.

Cholesterol Tests

Many cholesterol tests provide you with just a total cholesterol count and these are meaningless. Many patients with total cholesterol readings that are within safety levels could still be in great danger if that reading is mostly bad cholesterol LDL. The test must be able to give a separate reading of total and of bad cholesterol LDL and good cholesterol HDL levels. The recommended maximum level of LDL (bad cholesterol) is 3.0mmol.

The New Cholesterol Test

The new cholesterol test gives you the total cholesterol level and a separate reading of the HDL and the LDL. Only a pinprick drop of blood is required, like that used by diabetic patients to check their blood sugar levels. The patient is supplied with an easy-to-use extractor kit with full instructions. The drop of blood is returned in a specially prepared mini-tube and is then analysed at the laboratory. When the analysis is completed, the results will be posted to you. *(see example on page 60)*

This test requires a fasting blood sample. This small sample can easily be collected first thing in the morning in the privacy of your own home.

Everyone should have their cholesterol levels checked once every year. Cholesterol tests are not expensive and could safeguard you from one of the biggest killers in this country.

> **For details of how to order the new cholesterol test see Order Page at the back of this book.**

Cause of High Cholesterol

High cholesterol levels are associated with:
- Smoking
- Being overweight
- High blood presssure
- Lack of exercise
- Toxic gut

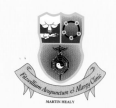

Example of Cholesterol Test Result

Name: Mr. XXX YYY
Address: XXXXX
            XXXX
            XXX

Test Date: 16th May 2007

Total Cholesterol
Total cholesterol level's should be less than   5.5 mmol/L
Your total cholesterol reading is   **5.0**

HDL (good cholesterol)
Good cholesterol level's should be higher than   1.2 mmol/L
Your good cholesterol reading is   **1.0**

LDL (bad cholesterol)
Bad cholesterol level's should be less than   3.0 mmol/L
Your bad cholesterol reading is   **4.0**

Laboratory Recommendation

Your total cholesterol levels are within the recommended range. However, your HDL is low and your LDL is above the recommended range.

It is imperative that you discuss these levels with your own GP and ask his advice.

LABORATORY REPORT

How to Treat High Cholesterol

For many people, their cholesterol levels will stabilise as they work to correct their causative factors.

High cholesterol levels are also associated with an unhealthy diet and an imbalance of friendly to unfriendly bacteria in the gut. There is now a significant body of evidence which suggests that high levels of friendly bacteria in the gut have the ability to metabolize (break down) cholesterol. It has been suggested that cholesterol may be a "food" for these friendly gut bacteria. This would explain how high levels of friendly gut bacteria often result in low levels of cholesterol in the blood.

This general theme of chronic disease stemming from bowel toxicity dates back to the work of Dr. Edward Bach (physician 1886 – 1936). He correctly stated that a dramatic improvement in health will be associated with the removal of these toxins.

(1) Use the Food Intolerance test as described in Chapter 12, to diagnose and remove the foods which are feeding these intestinal toxins.

(2) Too much saturated fat and trans fats can raise your LDL (bad cholesterol)

(3) Fried and fast food such as cakes, biscuits, pastry, chips, cream, fatty meats etc, are generally high in unhealthy fats.

(4) Increase your intake of fruit, vegetables and oily fish to help lower this bad cholesterol.

(5) Always discuss your cholesterol levels with your doctor as medication may be required in certain individual cases.

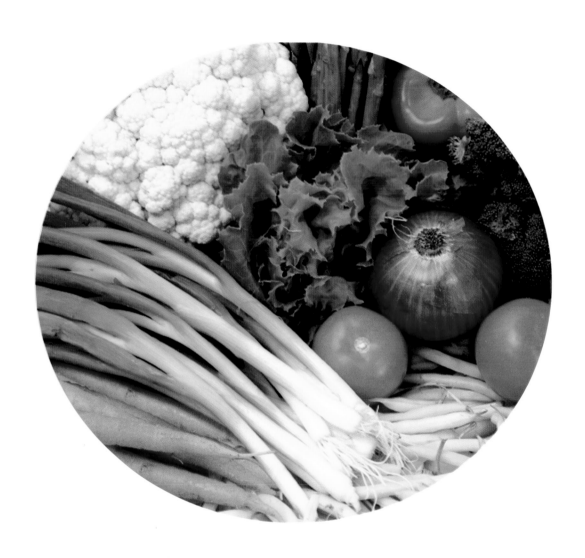

CHAPTER 12
ALLERGY TESTS

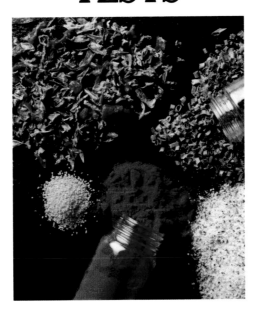

Introduction

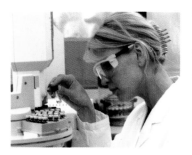

There are many kinds of allergy tests available. In order for an allergy testing approach to be viable and useful it should fulfil certain criteria:

- The test should be objective, not subject to human interpretation as this can lead to results which are influenced by the tester's own bias or beliefs.

- The test must be reproducible. This means that if the same person's blood is submitted several times, it should give the same result each time.

- The test should be able to grade the degree of allergy reaction. People who have food intolerance problems generally have two or three primary allergies, along with a small number of secondary allergies. Avoidance of the primary allergies alone is generally sufficient to resolve the problem.

*The 'Fitzwilliam **FoodCheck**' Food Intolerance Test*

A significant number of years have gone into researching, trialling and adjusting the test in collaboration with leading scientists in this area. It is only in the clinic context that I have been able to establish the exact test levels which signify a negative, minor or major reaction to the food. Within the clinic context, I have developed a number of procedures to ensure that the test is 100% accurate at all times. These procedures include random sampling, split sample trials and random and anonymous retesting of clients whose food sensitivities are well established.

Having been involved with allergy and food intolerance testing since 1983, and having worked with nearly every test which is available, I am convinced that the 'Fitzwilliam **FoodCheck**' test is the best and most useful tool currently available.

The 'Fitzwilliam *FoodCheck'* Test

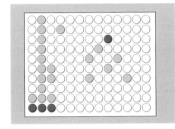

Another great advantage of the test is that it can be conducted in the person's own home. Only a pinprick drop of blood is required, like that used by diabetics to check their bloodsugar levels. The patient is supplied with an easy-to-use extractor kit with full instructions. The drop of blood is returned in a specially prepared container and is then analysed at the laboratory. When the analysis is completed the results will be posted to you.

The laboratory analysis involves specially designed test plates which have small wells on the surface. The most problematic foods are cultured in the wells and the patient's blood spread across the plate. If the blood contains immune cells which are antagonistic to a particular food, they will attach themselves to the inside of that well. After a set period of time, the plate is washed clean of all remaining blood particles. A special coloured dye is then added. This binds with the positive cells on the plate. The deeper the colour of the end product, the greater the degree of positive reaction.

It is important to note that the test only works on foods which have been consumed within three months prior to taking the blood sample, so it is important to eat a good cross-section of foods, especially the foods which you specifically want to have investigated, before taking the test.

> **For details of how to order the new 'Fitzwilliam FoodCheck' Food Intolerance test, see order page at the back of this book.**

Other Allergy Tests

It is my belief that the intolerance test is the best available for identifying slow response food allergies. There are, however, many others currently available, and their merits and disadvantages are discussed below.

The Prick & Scratch Method

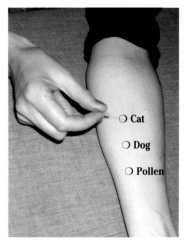

The first allergy test to be used by Western medical practitioners was the prick and scratch method and that is still the standard hospital test today. It was introduced around 1911 and has not developed much since then. A small drop of the substance being tested is dropped onto the skin, which is then either scratched or pricked with a needle. The amount of inflammation which develops at the scratch site indicates how allergic the substance is. This test is inaccurate when applied for the detection of the majority of food allergies and intolerances and gives many false readings. The prick and scratch method seems to work better when testing for external factors, such as dust, animal hair etc and for IgE reactions.

Patch Testing

A similar technique used in hospitals is patch testing. Small quantities of suspected substances are placed under individual cups which are then taped to the skin for a number of hours. A reddening of the skin under the patch denotes a sensitivity to that particular substance.

As with the prick and scratch method the patch test is perhaps more appropriate for testing external agents but is almost useless for checking for food allergies. Foods and other substances which are well-known by the individual to cause real reactions commonly fail to react with this test.

Cytotoxic Testing

This is a laboratory test in which the white blood cells are separated by centrifuge. They are then placed on a slide and the foods to be tested are added. A laboratory technician records the effects on the blood cells. The dependence on human interpretation is a major weakness, especially when multiple samples have to be monitored. The test was first introduced into the UK in the 1950s with a claim of 80% accuracy. It is currently in disrepute because of an inability to duplicate the findings from one laboratory to another, or even within the same laboratory on different runs.

The RAST Test

The RAST Test (radioimmunoassay) is another blood allergy test designed to detect the presence of IgE. In the case of foods, the value of the RAST test is limited, not because of its validity but because it measures only IgE, which accounts for only a small proportion of the food hypersensitivity picture.

Vega Testing

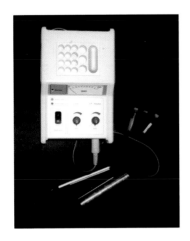

The Vega machine (known in the US as the Dermatron) is a very sensitive piece of electronic equipment used for measuring comparative resistance. The patient is given an electrode, which acts as an earth, to hold in one hand. A second electrode, designed as a probe, is brought in contact with one of the acupuncture points on the hand. Built into the Vega machine is an ammeter, which crosses the circuit. A special homeopathic allergy test ampoule is then introduced into the circuit and the degree of allergy is interpreted by assessing the degree of distortion recorded on the ammeter.

My personal opinion is that this machine is very difficult to use. Because of the extreme sensitivity of the machine it is almost impossible to get consistent readings and as a result its record of reproducibility is very poor. It is also totally subject to human interpretation. In addition, the final reading is affected by other factors, including the difficulty in achieving the correct angle or pressure with the probe, the friction it creates and the degree of moisture as a result of perspiration. These factors render the Vega machine unreliable in the diagnosis of food allergies.

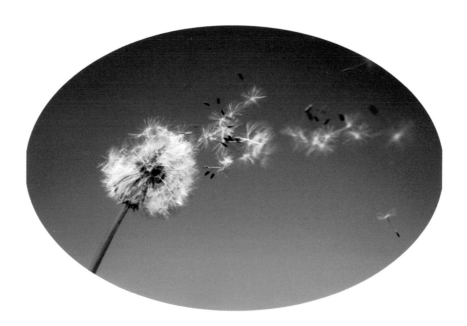

CHAPTER 13
THE THYROID -
(WEIGHT GAIN CONNECTION)

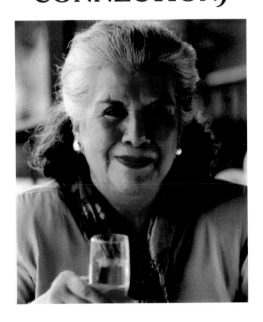

Introduction

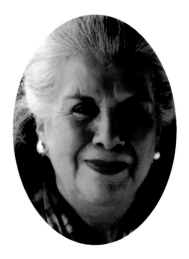

Most people who have difficulty loosing weight have an underlying thyroid problem. The thyroid gland produces a hormone called thyroxine and one of its vital functions is to control metabolism. In this context metabolism means the rate at which the body processes, utilises and then eliminates the waste products of the food which we eat. People with low thyroxine levels (hypothyroidism), will suffer chronic overweight problems, amongst other difficulties.

For reasons which are unclear, thyroid problems are becoming increasingly common. Some experts in this field estimate that up to 20% of the population suffer with thyroid problems. In addition to controlling metabolism, thyroxine provides that spark for the effective functioning of many of the body's vital life support systems. As a result, malfunction of the thyroid gland will reflect upon all of these vital body systems.

The Thyroid – food intolerance connection

What is becoming increasingly clear is that the majority of people who suffer with thyroid disease also suffer from food intolerance. The two are intimately connected.

Hyperthyroidism

Hyperthyroidism or excessive thyroxine production is relatively easy to diagnose. The excessive thyroxine hormone accelerates metabolism and all of the body systems. The diagnostic symptoms reflect this uncontrolled acceleration:

- Rapid weight loss
- Palpitations (rapid heartbeat)
- Irritability and nervousness
- Goitre (enlargement of the thyroid gland)
- Eye staring or bulging of eyes in socket

Hypothyroidism

Hypothyroidism or low thyroxine production is much more common but mostly goes undiagnosed. This is because the hypothyroidism develops slowly over an extended period of time and when tested for, the diagnostic laboratory tests frequently miss it.

The diagnostic symptoms are:

- Weight gain
- Fatigue
- Cold and constipation
- Depression and anxiety
- Headaches
- Skin and hair quality affected
- High cholesterol

These are the most important symptoms but there are many more. Thyroxine is required by all of the vital body systems including the immune system. The connection with weight gain and lack of energy is legendary. The depression connection stems from the fact that brain neurotransmitters which maintain mood stability, are unable to function in the absence of thyroxine. Tests for cholesterol in patients with thyroid problems always show it to be elevated. Once the thyroid is successfully treated, the cholesterol levels normalise.

Diagnosis

Hypothyroidism is much the bigger problem and it mostly goes undiagnosed, creeping up on individuals slowly and insidiously. The reason it goes undiagnosed is because the alarm bells ring loudest in the other body systems which suffer as a result of low thyroxine levels. The depression or exhaustion or intense headaches or chronic weight gain etc, are so distressing that they become the focus of attention. Very often the treatment focus is directed towards treating the depression or the headaches or whatever, and all the time the underlying thyroid disease remains undiagnosed. The other reason hypothyroidism goes undiagnosed is because the standard laboratory blood tests often allow the disease to become well established before confirming a diagnosis.

Laboratory Blood Tests

What is needed is a test which acts as an early warning system. This is exactly what the new Thyroid Antibody Test does.

Thyroid Antibody Test

Thyroid disease is typically a malfunction where the immune system destroys or over-stimulates thyroid tissue. It is almost always caused by the autoimmune condition Hishimoto's Thyroiditis, in which the body's immune system produces antibodies which attack the thyroid gland gradually making it inactive and causing hypothyroidism, or by Grave's Disease where the production of thyroid hormone is stimulated causing hyperthyroidism. This disease process where the body attacks its own organs is explained on page 18.

This new thyroid antibody test is able to detect these antibodies sent out by the immune system to attack the thyroid gland. Early detection of raised thyroid antibody levels can often precede the onset of symptoms by a year or more. The presence of these antibodies unequivocally confirms the diagnosis of thyroid disease.

Details of the Thyroid Antibody Test

Only a pinprick drop of blood is required, like that used by a diabetic patient to check their blood sugar levels. The patient is supplied with an easy-to-use extractor kit and full instructions. The few drops of blood are returned in a specially prepared mini-tube and is then analysed at the laboratory. When the analysis is completed, the result will be posted to you.

> For details of how to access the Thyroid Antibody Test see Order Page at the back of this book.

CHAPTER 14
WEIGHT-LOSS WITH THE GI DIET

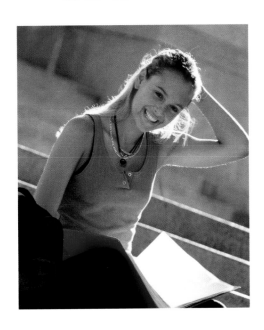

Introduction

People need to remember that their is a strong connection between thyroid malfunction and chronic overweight problems. Thyroid disease will block and stop you reaping any benefits from your dieting efforts. Thyroid details are explained in previous chapter.

The GI diet

The body turns the food that we eat into sugar (glucose) which is its source of energy. This glucose flows throughout the body in the bloodstream. This sugar powers our muscles to keep us going throughout the day. It also powers all of our body systems to keep them working for us. However, the glucose levels in the bloodstream has to be kept within a strict range. The blood glucose levels are constantly monitored and are kept within this strict range by the hormone insulin. If the blood glucose levels rise, the body releases insulin which stores away this excess sugar as fat. This is stored in the fat cells around your body.

The Principe of The GI Diet

When blood sugar levels are low, you feel hungry and crave food. However, the key to this new diet centres around the fact that certain foods cause a rapid increase in blood sugar levels. It is **this rapid rise** in blood sugar levels which triggers the insulin production and causes you to store this sugar rush as tissue fat. To loose weight you must stabilise your blood sugar levels. A slow steady increase in blood sugar levels does not trigger insulin production. The GI diet is based upon the principle of eating specific foods which raise your blood sugar levels, very slowly. The GI diet tells you which foods to eat and which foods to avoid.

The Atkins Diet

The Atkins Diet was relatively successful but controversial and is not recommended by this author. It was successful however, because it stabilised blood sugar levels. The GI diet as recommended here is even more successful and without all of the negative side effects associated with Atkins.

GI stands for Glycaemic Index

The index scores individual foods and the score tells us how quickly specific foods raise your blood sugar levels. The higher the score, the greater the sugar rush the food will give you. By choosing foods with a low GI, you are eating foods that digest and convert to sugar very slowly. They keep you feeling full for longer and this dramatically reduces the desire for more food. Most importantly of all, they stabilise your blood sugar and insulin levels.

For a complete food list refer to the coloured **GI index**. The index is divide into green, yellow and red columns. Foods in the green column are the good foods and have a low GI rating. Foods in the yellow column have a medium rating. Foods in the red column are bad because they have a high GI rating. To loose weight it is very simple, all you have to do is eat foods in the green column and avoid foods in the red column.

Additional Factors That Influence Blood Sugar levels

In addition to avoiding red column foods and only eating green column foods, there are additional factors which will influence your new improved healthy eating plan. Some of these additional factors are listed.

1. Protein

Incorporate protein into each meal as it slows the rate of conversion of the entire meal into glucose which helps to keep the blood glucose levels even. Protein will make you feel full for longer reducing the temptation to snack.

Proteins can be classified as (a) Heavy proteins and (b) Light proteins

Heavy proteins include skinless poultry. Fresh, frozen or tinned fish (never batter coated). Lean low-fat cuts of lamb which has been trimmed of all visible fat.

Light Proteins include goats cheese and yoghurt. Sheep's cheese and yoghurt. All soya products such as soya milk, yoghurt, tofu etc. Nuts, beans and lentils and products made from these are all regarded as light protein. Cow's milk skimmed is also a useful light protein.

Eat only one heavy protein meal in the day but ensure to incorporate a light protein food in every other meal and snack. Again the reason for incorporating protein is to slow the conversion of the meal into glucose.

2. Fat

Hydrogenated fats and oils must be avoided. Hydrogenated oils are vegetable oils which have been heat treated. In addition to bloating the fat cells they are a toxic irritant to the tissues and cause fluid retention. Many fast foods and snack foods including biscuits, cakes, muffins, pastry etc, contain hydrogenated oils. Check labels carefully.

The best fats are polyunsaturated and monounsaturated fats which have not been heat treated. Watch for non-hydrogenated fat on labels. Most vegetable oils such as corn, sunflower, olive, rapeseed etc, are ideal polyunsaturated oils.

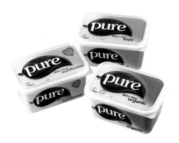

Fish oils also come highly recommended as they contain the essential omega-3 and 6 ingredients. Oily fish (tinned or fresh) such as salmon, tuna, sardines, mackerel etc, are all a very good source. *Pure* spread is another excellent product. It does not contain hydrogenated oils but uses polyunsaturated and monounsaturated oils. Pure Sunflower spread contains omega 3 and 6 and is a vegetarian source from Linseed Oil.

3. Food Intolerance Reactions

Food intolerance has an important role to play in chronic overweight problems. Food intolerance causes fluid retention and the best results are achieved when such foods are also removed. Some low GI foods, rank high on the list of the most common allergy / intolerant foods. If you fail to make progress on the GI diet, food intolerance is the most likely cause.

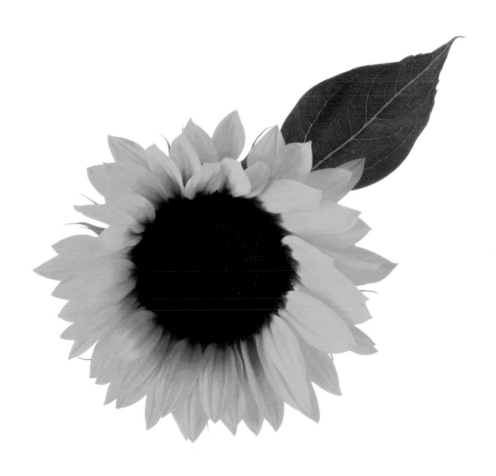

High GI Foods	Moderate GI Foods	Low GI Food
Mashed Potato 70	Muesli 56	Brocolli 10
White bread 70	Boiled potatoes 56	Cabbage 10
Cereals sugared 70	Sultanas 56	Garlic 10
Chocolate bars 70	Pitta bread 57	Green veg 10
Cola drinks 70	Basmati rice 58	Salted peanuts 14
Sugar 70	Honey 58	Low fat yoghurt 14
Watermelon 72	Digestive biscuites 59	Apricots - fresh 20
Swede 72	Cheese pizza 60	Grapefruit 20
Begel 72	Ice cream 61	Cherries 22
Branflakes 74	New potatoes 62	Green lentils 22
Cheerios 74	Apricots tinned 64	Dark cocoa choc 22
Waffles 76	Raisins 64	Grapefruit 25
Coco pops 77	Shortbread biscuits 64	Red lentils 26
Water biscuits 78	Couscous 65	Whole milk 27
Jelly beans 80	Rye bread 65	All bran 30
Crackers 80	Banana 65	Apple 30
Potato crisps 80	Pineapple 66	Beans 30
Rice cakes 82	Croissants 67	Peas 30
Rice Krispies 82	Shredded wheat 67	Dried apricots 31
Cornflakes 84	Mars bar 68	Skimmed milk 32
Jacket Potato 85	Ryvita 69	Apricots - dried 35
Carrots (cooked) 85	Weetabix 69	Carrots - raw 35
Popcorn 85		Brown Spaghetti 37
Puffed wheat 89		Apples 38
Potato mashed 90		Pears 38
Rice pre-cooked 90		Canned soup 38
Baguette 95		Bread unrefined 40
Lucozade 95		Spaghetti unrefin 40
Potato chips 95		All bran 42
Parsnips boiled 97		Porridge 42
White rice steamed 98		Baked beans 48
Beer 110		Wholemeal bread 53

CHAPTER 15
FIVE ELEMENT ACUPUNCTURE

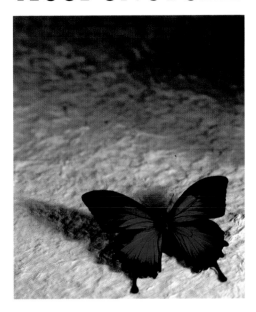

Introduction

In addition to avoiding your culprit foods it is also helpful to strengthen the digestive system. As has been repeatedly said throughout this book, factors such as stress, worry, anxiety etc, are the primary triggers of food intolerance symptoms. The digestive system has a direct nerve supply and through these nerves, digestive "health" is severely affected in times of stress. People who suffer from food intolerance problems tend to lock this stress within their nervous system. It is often the case that they find it very difficult to relax. This nervous energy needs to be drained away and a treatment applied which will relax and calm the entire nervous system. Acupuncture is one of the fastest and most powerful ways of clearing this blocked nervous energy and resetting the entire digestive system. Perhaps you should consider having a course of acupuncture.

Background

Acupuncture has been practised in China for at least 2,000 years. The practice spread to other countries of the Orient and, as it did, individual interpretations and styles of application began to emerge.

Five Element Acupuncture

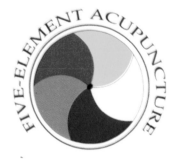

One of the first and one of the most influential masters of classical acupuncture in the West was Professor J.R. Worsley.

Professor J.R. Worsley

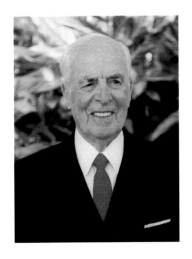

A style of acupuncture which specifically focuses upon the worries and stresses of the patient has become known as Five Element Acupuncture, and one man who did more than any to bring this particular style to the Western world is Professor J.R. Worsley. Worsley is an Englishman who studied acupuncture in the early '60s in Taiwan and other parts of the Far East. After he returned from the East, he founded the College of Traditional Acupuncture in England to teach this style of treatment.

I studied with Professor Worsley at the UK College of Traditional Acupuncture from 1980 to 1983.

Worsley's emphasis runs in tandem with other Western physicians of the last century who were developing treatment systems which were focused upon the stressed and worried emotions of their patients. Most influential in this work was the German homeopath and physician Dr. Samuel Hahnemann, and the English herbalist and physician Dr. Edward Bach.

There are many different styles of acupuncture, each with a different emphasis. It is not that any one is superior to the others as different styles suit different conditions, but I believe that the Five Element style, as taught by Worsley, is particularly appropriate for people who have allergies.

What to expect when attending an Acupuncture Practitioner

The Five Element acupuncture approach aims to release the nervous energy which has become blocked within the nervous system. It also has the potential to strengthen it, and thus enable it to resist future emotional stresses more efficiently. As a result of treatment, people feel emotionally stronger within themselves. They are uplifted and generally better able to cope with life. As the nervous system relaxes, the immune system stops producing allergy reactions.

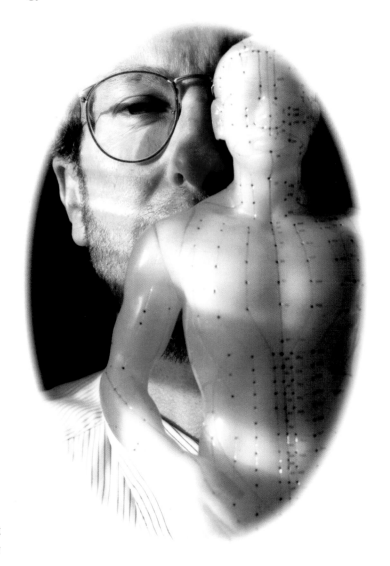

Photos courtesy of Frank
Miller, *The Irish Times*

CHAPTER 16
CONCLUSION

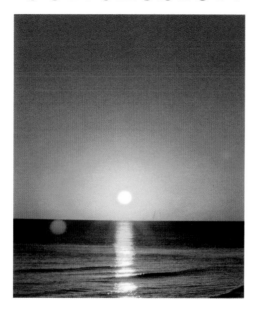

Conclusion

Sorting out your health is not impossible and it does not have to cost the earth. If you have a food intolerance problem, find out what that intolerance is. Most people have relatively few primary intolerances and the detection and avoidance of these foods is sufficient to bring about a dramatic recovery in health.

The irony of it all is that many of you, who perhaps sat at your breakfast table this morning, demoralised as a result of your present medical condition, bewildered as a result of the utter failure of science to ease your plight, at a complete loss as to what you should do next, will be very surprised to find that the cause of all your distress has been on that plate in front of you, looking at you straight in the face.

Martin Healy

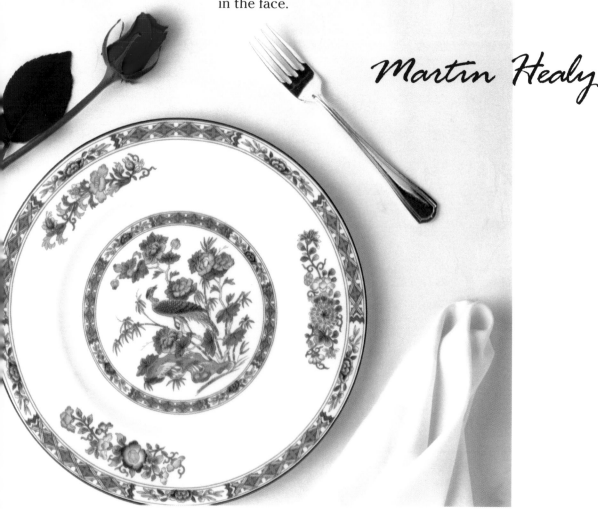

INDEX

Test Order Page (PHOTOCOPIABLE)

To order a test you have three options

A   Phone the clinic on 01 4733790 and quote your credit card number. Your order will then be posted directly to you.

B   Write to the clinic indicating your requirement and post it with appropropriate payment. Your order will then be posted directly to you.
(Make sure to include your full postal address and contact telephone number)

C   Email the clinic at fitzwil@gmail.com

Please make check payable to:
Fitzwilliam Clinic

and post to:
Fitzwilliam Clinic
114 Herberton Road,
South Circular Road
Dublin 8
Ireland

1. The 'Fitzwilliam **Food*Check*'** Food intolerance Test. . . €255

2. Saliva Hormone Test €125

3. Cholesterol Test €85

4. Thyroid Antibody Test €95

5. Osteoporosis Test €85

Note: The **Food*Check*** Food Intolerance Test is also available from select Sam McCauley Chemist outlets.